Keto Fat Bombs In Under 10 Minutes

Sweet and Savory Snacks For Weight Loss

Rick Elliott

Text Copyright © 2018 Rick Elliott

All rights reserved. No part of this guide may be reproduced in any form without permission in writing from the publisher except in the case of brief quotations embodied in critical articles or reviews.

Legal & Disclaimer

The information contained in this book and its contents is not designed to replace or take the place of any form of medical or professional advice; and is not meant to replace the need for independent medical, financial, legal or other professional advice or services, as may be required. The content and information in this book has been provided for educational and entertainment purposes only.

The content and information contained in this book has been compiled from sources deemed reliable, and it is accurate to the best of the Author's knowledge, information and belief. However, the Author cannot guarantee its accuracy and validity and cannot be held liable for any errors and/or omissions. Further, changes are periodically made to this book as and when needed. Where appropriate and/or necessary, you must consult a professional (including but not limited to your doctor, attorney, financial advisor or such other professional advisor) before using any of the suggested remedies, techniques, or information in this book.

Upon using the contents and information contained in this book, you agree to hold harmless the Author from and against any damages, costs, and expenses, including any legal fees potentially resulting from the application of any of the information provided by this book. This disclaimer applies to any loss, damages or injury caused by the use and application, whether directly or indirectly, of any advice or information presented, whether for breach of contract, tort, negligence, personal injury, criminal intent, or under any other cause of action.

You agree to accept all risks of using the information presented inside this book.

You agree that by continuing to read this book, where appropriate and/or necessary, you shall consult a professional (including but not limited to your doctor, attorney, or financial advisor or such other advisor as needed) before using any of the suggested remedies, techniques, or information in this book.

Legal & Disclaimer

Contents

Introduction

Thousands of people typically try to avoid food rich in fat owing to the misconception that these are main culprits responsible of packing in unwanted pounds. For those who are unaware of the keto diet, it's all about minimizing your carbohydrate intake and eating more fats. After time on the diet, your body goes into ketosis. That means your cells don't have enough carbohydrates to use for energy, so your body creates ketones and burns fat instead. If you decide to stick to this low-carb diet, then note that around 70 to 80 percent of your calorie intake every day should be derived from fat. Around 15 to 20 percent should be dedicated to protein while the remaining 5 percent should come from carbs.

While this is a big change from what often people told you to eat, it arguably plays a major part in attaining your weight loss goals, provided stick strictly to the guidelines. You may also have been introduced to the keto fat bombs, the favorite go-to snacks of the proponents of this diet plan. Think of these fat bombs as energy balls. The only difference is that they do not fully depend on carbs to as a major nutrient of these energy treats.

What the fat bombs contain, instead, are fat. In most cases, they are made of 80 percent fat. These them handy choices for your quick breakfast, afternoon treats, or post or pre-workout snacks.. Even if you are not following the keto diet religiously, it is still possible for you to enjoy the wonders and tastes of these fat bombs. A bonus treat is since it is mostly fat, your digestive tract breaks it down more slowly, so expect the bombs to make you feel full for a far longer time.

Keen to know how to go about making easy keto fat bombs? In fact, most of them you can even make under 10 minutes, with the help of this book.

Chapter 1 – Why Make Keto Fat Bombs?

Fat bombs refer to small, high-fat and low-carb treats that are popular among those who are following the ketogenic diet. These treats serve as replacement meals or as fun and delicious snacks. If you are interested in these treats, then I'm sure that you will be happy to know that you have the choice between making them savory or sweet. Keto fat bombs are also known for being loaded with fats, so expect them to be capable of curbing your appetite while boosting your metabolism.

Fat bombs are capable of providing an additional boost of energy for those who are planning to work out and also to replace lost energy after your workout. They even have the ability to fight your cravings for a few extra hours. In addition, they can satisfy your taste buds so you won't feel deprived, especially if you are on a diet.

One thing to take note of when planning to eat fat bombs for weight loss is to make them a part of your low-carb diet. You can't expect them to perform their job if you fill your body with too much carbs. What you should do is to eat the fat bombs once every day either as a fun snack or as a means of leveling up the amount of healthy fats your diet contains.

A lot of people consume one fat bomb for either breakfast or lunch, and they say that it is already enough to make them full for hours. It is definitely effective in curbing your hunger and aiding in weight loss.

Nutrition

Fat bombs contain a lot of fat, but the good news is that the ketogenic recipes in this book only consists of healthy or 'good fat'. You need the good fats for your body to function well. In fact, your daily calorie intake should have at least 20% good fat.

These good fats are necessary for absorbing fat-soluble vitamins, such as Vitamins A, D, E, and K. Examples are monounsaturated fats, or those that you can find in olives, peanuts, and avocados, can lower your bad cholesterol and increase the amount of good one. It also takes longer for your digestive tract to break down good fats. Furthermore, it is capable of slowing down the process of breaking down carbs into sugar, which is a major help in stabilizing your blood sugar levels.

They are also designed to help you stay full for a longer period. In fact, one spoon of coconut oil daily can trim down your waistline. Keeping those benefits in mind, you definitely have enough reasons to really start making fat bombs a part of your diet. Just make sure to continue watching your portion sizes. Taking in a fat bomb during breakfast is a major help if you want to prevent yourself from snacking.

The nutritional benefits of fat bombs can be categorized into the following:

- Allows your body to absorb various fat-soluble vitamins, like Vitamins A, D, and E

- Lowers bad cholesterol while increasing the good by ensuring that the fat bomb is made out of olives, peanuts, and other sources of healthy fats

- Slows down your digestion as well as the breakdown of carbs to sugar – This not only stabilizes your blood sugar level but also helps you stay fuller for a longer period. You can, therefore, prevent overeating and binge snacking.

- Accelerates weight loss – It is mainly because of the coconut oil used in making the fat bomb.

Chapter 2 – The Basics of Making Keto Fat Bombs

Fat bombs are considered as flavorful combinations of ketogenic ingredients. You can enjoy them not only as snacks and desserts, but also as meal replacements. All fat bombs contain more than 90% fat. What's good about them is that you can easily make them. There are even various flavors to choose from.

Decide on the textures and flavors

Before you can make a fat bomb, you have to know exactly the kind of flavor you prefer. Note that there are several flavors that you can incorporate into this food. You can make it sweet, crunchy, spicy, cheesy, savory, bitter, or sour. Decide on a specific flavor or flavor combination you want to attain as this is what will help you make the most satisfying keto fat bombs.

Determine your fat base

All fat bombs need a fat base, which is crucial in solidifying the foods when you refrigerate them. The fat base also helps the fat bombs stay solid when you put them at room temperature. Among the most reliable and commonly used fat bases are butter and coconut oil. If you are choosing butter, then ensure that you go for the 100% grass-fed one.

You can also use cream cheese. Furthermore, there are other less commonly used fat bases that you can experiment on. You can use animal fats, such as tallow, for instance. Another option is to try to reform and melt cheese together with your keto ingredients.

Prepare the other keto ingredients

After figuring out the best fat base that you can use, check your cupboard or visit a store to find more ingredients that you can incorporate into your recipes. Also, ensure that you have some of the most commonly used ingredients in these recipes.

These include salt, calorie-free sweeteners, such as sucralose, and powdered herbs and spices. You can also refer to the next chapter of this book to check the list of the most common ingredients that you need.

Combine them

Once you have the fat base and gathered some keto ingredients, you can finally combine them to create a delicious bar or ball. Do this by softening or melting the fat base first then blending or mixing the other ingredients. You can form the softened fat base into a bar or ball and refrigerate it.

The good news is that you can also choose to make your preferred shape. You can also transfer the melted fat base into a tray, plate, or container and refrigerate the bombs until they become solid.

The above-mentioned tips and steps are the basic ones. With that, you will notice just how simple it is to make fat bombs. The real challenge is in making them look good. One thing to remember though, is that you do not have to make your fat bombs look like rolled balls or candy pieces all the time. It is also possible to make them in various other forms, like mug cakes and cookies.

Chapter 3 – The Keto Fat Bomb Shopping List

- **Coconut oil** – This is the ideal fat that you can use in dessert and sweet fat bombs. However, it should not be the sole reason to include it in your shopping list. Another reason is that it is rich in medium-chain triglycerides. With that, taking even just a small amount of it, like a single tablespoon, can already help you reach ketosis.

- **High-fat dairy** – You also have to shop for high-fat dairy ingredients and include them in your recipes. Go for the 100% grass-fed one. Aside from being rich in CLA, an anti-inflammatory fatty acid, high-fat dairy can also provide you with fat-soluble vitamins, like Vitamins A, D, E, and K. It also has various amounts of Vitamin C and B-vitamins.

  Furthermore, high-fat dairy ingredients are rich in essential minerals, such as magnesium, zinc, phosphorus, selenium, potassium, and calcium. This will be a big help in replenishing the loss of minerals that's often one of the most common side effects of sticking to a keto diet.

- **Spices** – You also have to include spices in your shopping list. Aside from enhancing taste, you can also expect these spices to be good for your health in various ways. For instance, cinnamon is a spice, which is known for being a powerful immune system and antibacterial booster.

  You can also use clover, another spice rich in antibacterial and antioxidant properties. Add cloves and cinnamon into your next recipe to transform bland desserts into more savory treats.

- **Herbs** –What is good about herbs is that they are rich in antioxidants and essential vitamins and minerals. One example is fresh basil, which can enhance the taste of your savory pizza fat bomb recipes.

  You can also try adding rosemary into your fat bomb. This is another herb which adds flavor to your recipe. Aside from that, it can improve your cognitive function and make savory fat bombs even tastier.

- **Low-carb fruits** – It is also possible for you to incorporate fruits into your recipes but choose the low-carb ones, like blueberries and lemons. Also, ensure the fruits you add are truly healthy and can add more nutrients into your fat bombs apart from the flavors.

- **Low-carb veggie** – You can enjoy the fat bombs as meal replacements by adding a couple of low-carb veggies into them. You can add chives, for instance. You can also incorporate leafy greens as well as other healthy low-carb veggies. Incorporate the veggies together with your prepared fat bomb. For instance, you can make a veggie salad and place the fat bomb over it, so you can enjoy a more nutritious and satisfying meal.

- **Nuts and seeds** – Do not forget to shop for nuts and seeds too. What's good about these ingredients is that they can also supply the fiber, fat, and protein that are often lacking in the recipes. Some seeds that you can use are chia, sesame, and flax seeds. Nut butter or crushed nuts can also make your fat bombs even more satisfying, tasty, and nutritious.

Chapter 4 – Savory Keto Fat Bomb Recipes

Jalapeno Popper Fat Bombs

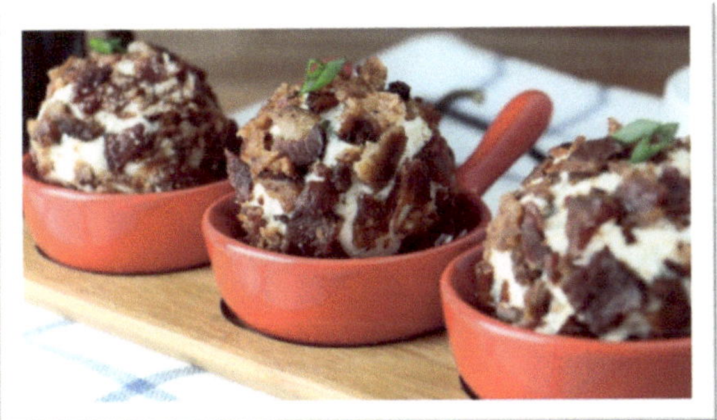

Ingredients:

- 3 slices of bacon

- 3-oz. cream cheese

- ½ tsp. dried parsley

- 1 medium-sized jalapeno pepper

- ¼ tsp. each of garlic powder and onion powder

- Salt and pepper

Instructions:

1. Fry the bacon slices in a pan until they turn crisp. Take the bacon out of the pan. Make sure to set aside the left grease in the pan for use later. Wait for a bit until the bacon is crisp and cool.

2. De-seed the jalapeno pepper. You should then dice it into tiny pieces.

3. Mix the spices, jalapeno pepper, and cream cheese in a bowl. Season it with some salt and pepper.

4. Add the reserved bacon fat or grease into the mixture. Combine them until you formed a solid mixture.

5. Crumble the bacon slices and put on a plate. Form balls out of the cream cheese mixture with the use of your hand. After that, you can roll each ball into the bacon.

Nutritional Value: Calories – 147; Net Carbs – 2.13 grams; Protein – 4.77 grams; Fat – 13.29 grams

Savory Salmon Fat Bombs

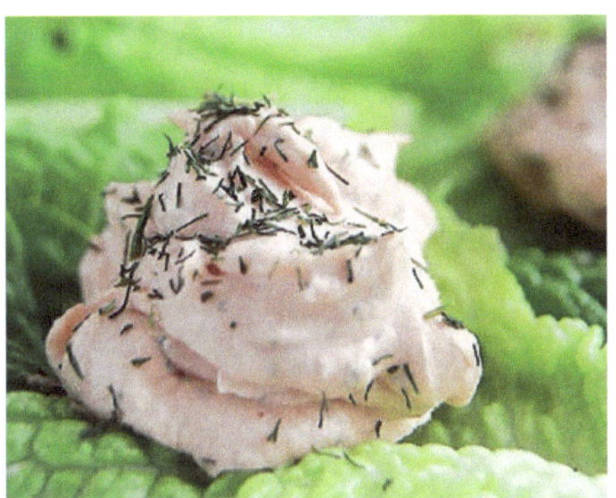

Ingredients:

- 1/3 cup grass-fed butter

- ½ cup full-fat cream cheese

- 1 tbsp. fresh lemon juice

- ½ pack smoked mackerel or salmon

- 1-2 tbsps. dill (freshly chopped)

Instructions:

1. Put the smoked salmon, butter, and cream cheese in your food processor. Add the dill and fresh lemon juice. Pulse the mixture until smooth.

2. Prepare a tray and line it with parchment paper. Start forming small fat bombs. Each bomb should use around two and one-half of the prepared mixture. Use dill as garnish and store in your fridge for a while to solidify.

3. Once solidified, serve right away.

Nutrition Value: Calories – 147; Net carbs – 0.7 grams; Protein – 3.2 grams; Fat – 15.7 grams

Bacon-wrapped Mozzarella Sticks

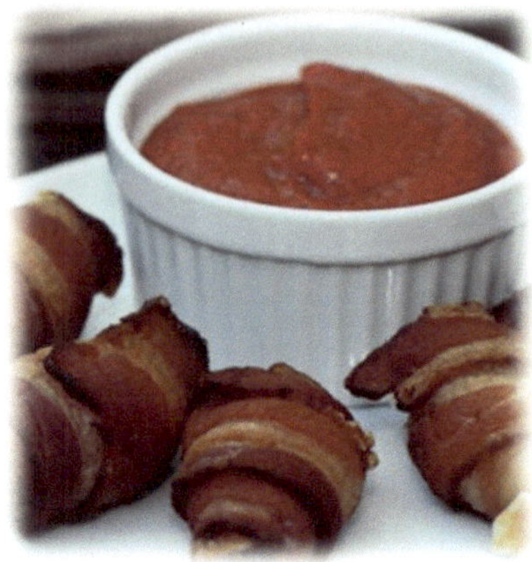

Ingredients:

- 2 bacon slices

- 1 mozzarella cheese stick – Cut it in half.

- Low-sugar pizza sauce (optional ingredient) – for dipping purposes

- Some coconut oil for frying

Instructions:

1. Preheat the coconut oil using your deep fryer.

2. Wrap the cheese sticks with bacon. Make sure to overlap while wrapping to ensure that the bacon stays intact. Use a toothpick to secure the wrapped cheese sticks.

3. Fry the bacon-wrapped cheese into the preheated oil. This should take around 2-3 minutes or until you notice that the bacon is crispy and brown.

4. Once done, transfer into a paper towel then let them cool for a while. Take the toothpick out and serve and enjoy together with your preferred dip.

Nutritional Value: Calories – 103; Net carbs – 1 gram per piece; Protein – 7 grams; Fat – 9 grams

Buffalo Chicken Deviled Eggs

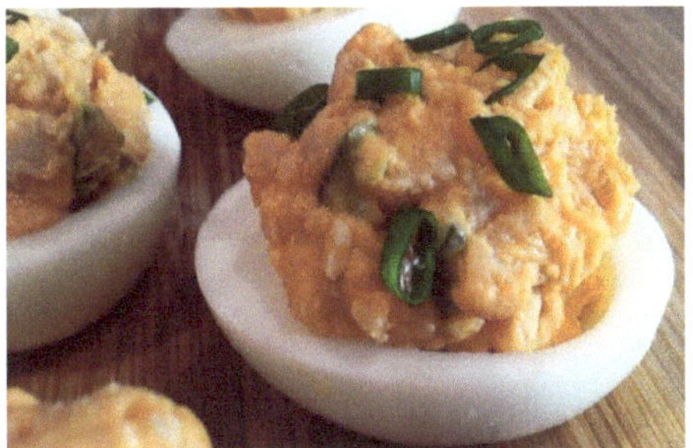

Ingredients:

- 6 large hard-boiled eggs

- ¼ of a small onion

- 6-oz. cooked and chopped chicken

- ¼ cup each of Franks Buffalo Wing sauce and blue cheese crumbles

- 2 tbsps. blue cheese dressing

- Chopped small rib celery

Instructions:

1. Chop the celery and chicken while the eggs are still boiling.

2. After that, peel the hard-boiled eggs then cut them in half lengthwise. Get a large mixing bowl and scrape the egg yolks out and put in the bowl. Add the remaining ingredients into the bowl with the exception of the onion. What you have to do is to grate the onion using a micro-plane over the bowl. This is essential in ensuring that the onion's juice will add more flavor into the mixture.

3. Mix all the ingredients in the bowl. You should then put it into a zip-loc bag. Squeeze the added mixture into one of the corners of the zip-loc bag. Sniff off its corner. You should then use this in piping the mixture into the eggs.

Nutritional Value: Calories – 112; Net carbs – 1.3 grams; Protein – 7.5 grams; Fat – 8.5 grams

Bacon-wrapped Mini Meatloaves

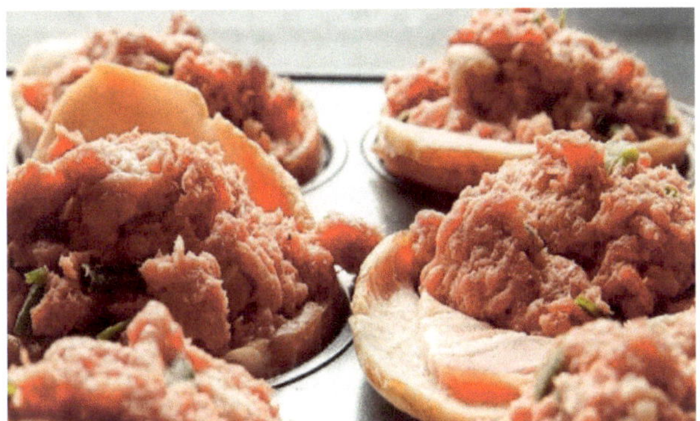

Ingredients:

- 1 lb. ground beef

- 1 additional bacon strips

- ½ lb. chunked bacon

- ¼ cup coconut milk

- 1/3 cup minced fresh chives

- 2 minced garlic cloves

- Chopped fresh parsley

- Freshly ground black pepper

Instructions:

1. Preheat oven.

2. Mix the bacon chunks, ground beef, chives, garlic, and coconut milk together in a bowl. Ensure that you mix well until all used ingredients hold together.

3. Use some freshly ground black pepper to season the mixture.

4. Get a medium-sized muffin tin. Put one bacon slice around the sides of every muffin tin hole. Fill the holes with the prepared beef mixture.

5. Put in your preheated oven and cook for around 20-30 minutes.

6. Take them out of the oven then wait for them to cool down. Once cool enough, you can take the mini-meatloaves out of the muffin tins.

7. Sprinkle the top with fresh parsley and serve.

Nutritional Value: Calories – 101; Carbs – 2 grams; Protein – 58 grams; Fat – 51 grams

Keto Butter Burgers

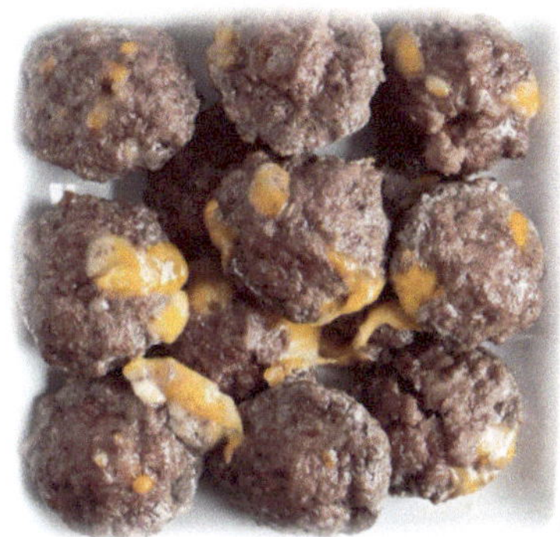

Ingredients:

- 1 lb. ground lean beef

- 3 tbsps. butter

- 2 oz. cheese

- Salt and pepper

- Onion powder and garlic powder (optional)

Instructions:

1. Preheat your oven.

2. Mix the lean ground beef with your preferred amount of pepper and salt together in a bowl. Add garlic and onion powder if you are using.

3. Press some beef, around one tablespoon, at the bottom of a non-stick muffin pan. Make sure that the bottom part is completely covered.

4. Pat some butter on top of each beef. Add beef on top again. Press it to flatten.

5. The next step is to add a tiny piece of cheese on top. Put the last layer of beef then press to flatten. Bake in your oven for around 10 minutes.

6. You should remove each one from the pan and put on a plate once cool enough to handle. Serve.

Nutritional Value: Calories – 125; Fat – 10 grams; Protein – 8 grams

Savory Sesame Fat Bombs

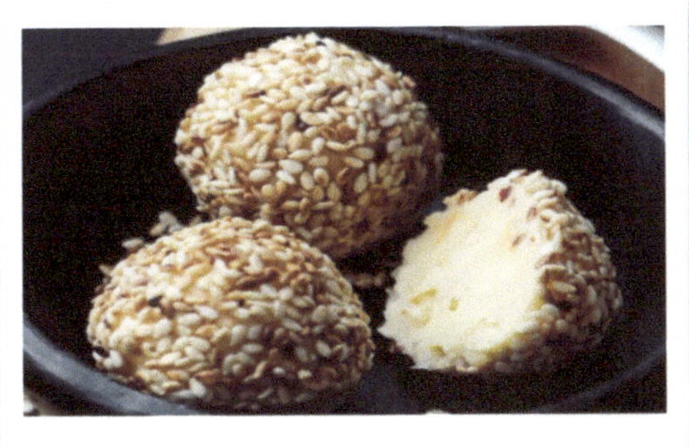

Ingredients:

- 4-oz. room temperature butter

- 1 tsp. sea salt

- 2 tbsps. sesame oil

- 2 tsps. toasted sesame seeds

- ¼ tsp. chili flakes

Instructions:

1. Roast the sesame seeds for a few minutes in a hot and dry pan. Ensure that you don't burn them. You know that they're done if they turn to golden brown and begin to pop. Transfer to a shallow bowl or plate immediately. Set aside.

2. Mix salt, chili flakes, sesame oil, and butter in a bowl. Store in your fridge for a while to solidify.

3. After that, you should start shaping balls from the butter mixture then roll each one in the sesame seeds you've toasted earlier. Store in your fridge to firm up before serving.

Nutritional Value: Calories – 272; Net carbs – 0.2 grams; Protein – 1 gram; Fat – 30 grams

Olives and Cheese Savory Fat Bombs

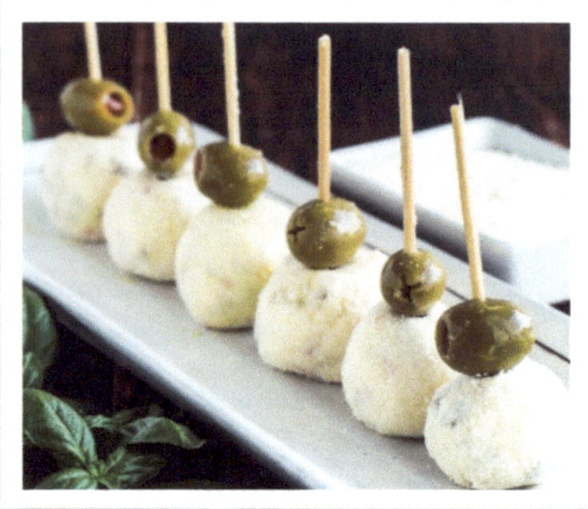

Ingredients:

- 5-oz. cream cheese

- 6 chopped olives

- 1 tsp. minced garlic

- 2 tbsps. parmesan cheese

- ¼ tsp. salt

Instructions:

1. Mix together the garlic, salt, chopped olives and cream cheese in a bowl. Continue mixing until well combined.

2. Scoop balls out of the mixture then put in your fridge to let them harden a bit prior to rolling them.

3. Sprinkle parmesan cheese over a plate then roll the formed cream cheese balls into it until they are fully covered.

4. Store in your fridge until you are ready to serve them.

Nutritional Value: Calories – 75; Carbs – 1 gram; Protein – 2 grams; Fats – 7 grams

Baked Brie and Pecan Fat Bomb

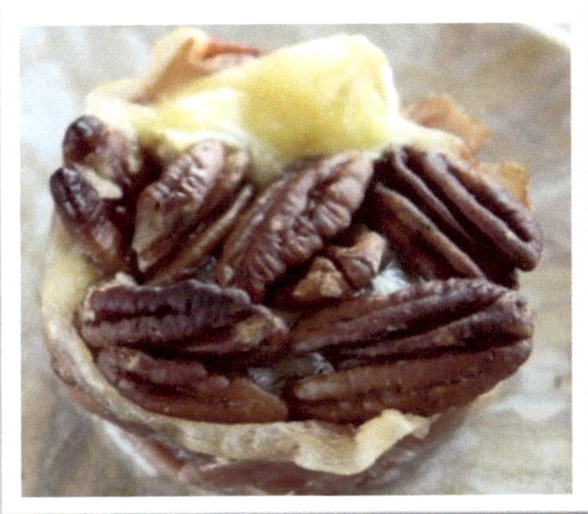

Ingredients:

- 1-oz. full-fat Brie cheese

- 1 slice prosciutto

- 1/8 tsp. black pepper

- 6 pecan halves

Instructions:

1. Preheat your oven. Prepare a muffin tin, too.

2. Get the slice of prosciutto. Fold this slice in half to make it almost square.

3. Put it in the muffin tin's hole. Your goal is to line it completely.

4. Get the brie and chop it into small cubes. Ensure that you leave their white skin on. Put the chopped Brie into the cup lined with prosciutto.

5. The next thing to do is sticking the pecan halves among the brie.

6. Bake in your preheated oven until the brie melts and the prosciutto is already cooked. Allow it to cool for a while before taking it out of the muffin pan.

Nutritional Value: Calories – 183; Net carbs – 0.43 grams; Protein – 8.42 grams; Fat – 16 grams

Stuffed Pecan Fat Bombs

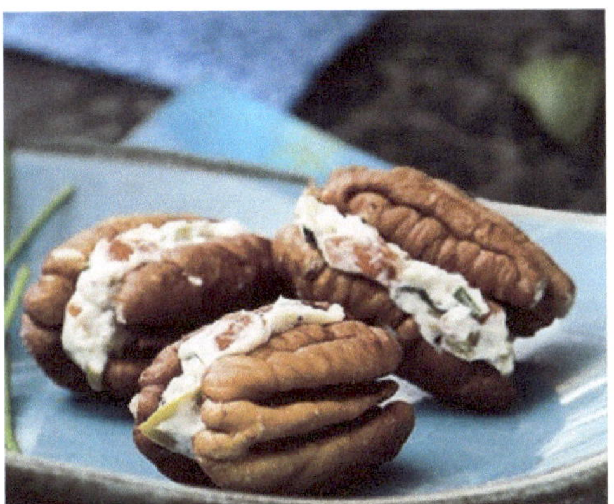

Ingredients:

- 4 pecan halves

- 1-oz. cream cheese

- ½ tsp. unsalted butter

- A pinch of salt

Instructions:

1. Toast the pecans in your oven. After toasting, set them aside and let them cool down for a while.

2. Soften the cream cheese and butter. You should then add your preferred flavor, herb, spice, or veggie. Combine well until a smooth and creamy mixture is attained.

3. Get two pecan halves and spread the cheese mixture in between them.

4. Sprinkle with some sea salt before serving.

Nutritional Value: Calories – 150; Carbs – 2 grams; Protein – 11 grams; Fat – 31 grams

Avocado and Chorizo Fat Bombs

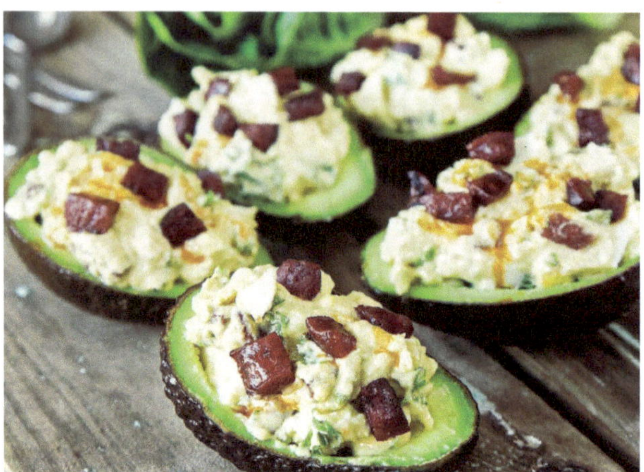

Ingredients:

- 3.5-oz. diced Spanish chorizo sausage

- 2 hardboiled eggs (peeled and diced)

- ¼ cup room temperature unsalted butter

- 2 tbsps. mayonnaise

- 2 tbsps. fresh chives (chopped)

- 1 tbsp. lemon juice (freshly squeezed)

- Cayenne pepper and salt

- 4 pitted avocado halves

Instructions:

1. Fry the chorizo in a heated pan until it becomes crispy. Once done, take it out of the heat then set aside for a while.

2. Mix the chorizo, eggs, and butter in a bowl. Use a fork to mash them together. Add chives, lemon juice, and mayonnaise. Use the salt and cayenne pepper as seasoning. Continue using the fork to combine the ingredients. Store in your fridge until it is set.

3. Prior to serving, top each half of avocado with a quarter of the chorizo and egg mixture. Serve right away.

Nutritional Value: Calories – 419; Net carbs – 2.7 grams; Protein – 11.4 grams; Fat – 38.9 grams

Keto Pistachio Truffles

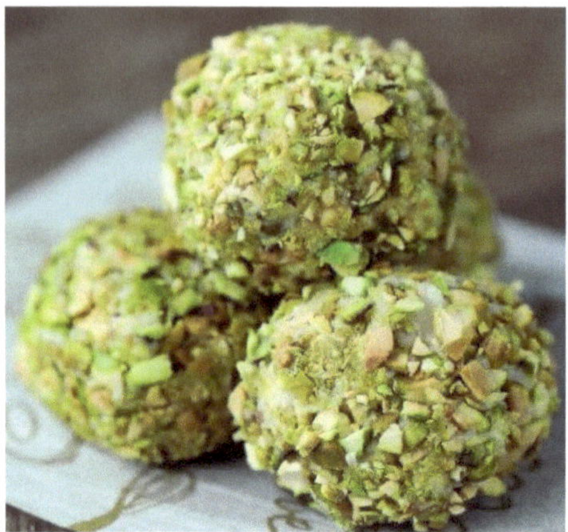

Ingredients:

- 8-oz. softened mascarpone cheese

- 3 tbsps. confectioner's style sweetener

- ¼ tsp. pure vanilla extract

- ¼ cup pistachios (chopped)

Instructions:

1. Mix vanilla, sweetener, and mascarpone together in a bowl. Use a spatula or fork to mix the ingredients gently yet thoroughly. Ensure that you create a smooth and well-blended mixture.

2. Form balls from the mixture using your hands. Each ball should be around one inch in diameter.

3. Put the pistachios in a small plate. Roll the truffles in the pistachios until coated completely. Store in your fridge for a while to chill prior to serving.

Nutritional Value: Calories – 121; Net carbs – 0.5 gram; Protein – 1 gram; Fat – 12 grams

Chapter 5 – Sweet Keto Fat Bomb Recipes

Macadamia Chocolate Fat Bombs

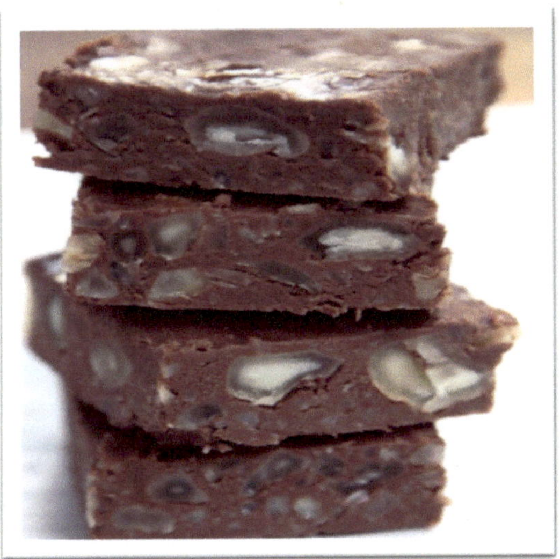

Ingredients:

- 2 oz. cocoa butter

- 2 tbsps. unsweetened cocoa powder

- 4 oz. chopped macadamia

- 2 tbsps. Swerve

- ¼ cup heavy cream

Instructions:

1. Melt the cocoa butter in a saucepan then add the cocoa powder. Stir in the Swerve. Mix together well until you produce a melted and well-blended mixture.

2. Add the chopped macadamias. Stir the mixture well.

3. Pour the cream then mix the ingredients again.

4. Pour the mixture into paper candy cups or molds. Allow them to cool then store in your refrigerator to let them harden a bit.

5. Serve and enjoy.

Nutritional Value: Calories – 267; Carbs – 3 grams; Protein – 3 grams; Fat – 28 grams

Chocolate and Coconut Cups

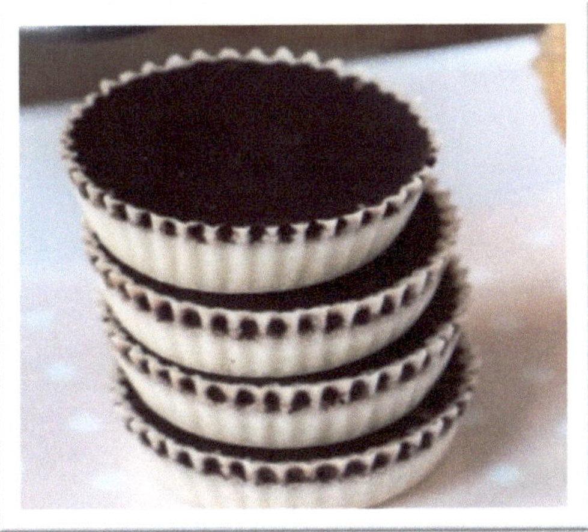

Ingredients:

- ¼ cup coconut butter

- 1 cup unsweetened coconut (shredded)

- ¼ cup coconut oil

- 1 tsp. vanilla extract

- 3-oz. 100% dark chocolate

- Stevia

Instructions:

1. Prepare a muffin pan and line it with a liner.

2. Put the coconut oil and coconut butter in a saucepan. Set it at low heat to soften the mentioned ingredients.

3. Add the shredded coconut into the mixture. Pour the vanilla extract and add the stevia. Mix well.

4.   Once done, divide the prepared mixture into the muffin cups. Place it in your refrigerator to let it set.

5.   The next step is melting the dark chocolate in your microwave or in a pan. Spoon it on top of each solid coconut cup. Put back in your fridge to set even further before serving.

Nutritional Value: Calories – 190; Carbs – 4 grams; Protein – 3 grams; Fat – 17 grams

Blueberry Cream Pie Fat Bomb

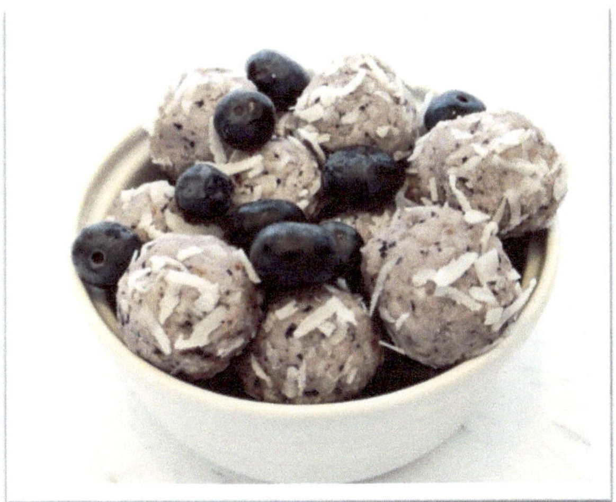

Ingredients:

- ½ cup blueberries

- 4 oz. soft goat cheese

- 1 tsp. vanilla extract

- 1 cup almond flour

- ½ tsp. stevia

- ½ cup pecans

- ¼ cup shredded coconut (unsweetened)

Instructions:

1. Use your food processor to process all the ingredients until everything is mixed.

2. Form small fat bombs from the processed mixture.

3.   Pour some coconut flakes in a bowl. Roll each of the formed fat bombs lightly into the shredded coconut.

4.   Serve.

Nutritional Value: Calories – 48; Carbs – 1 gram; Protein – 1 gram; Fat – 4 grams

Pumpkin Pie Patties

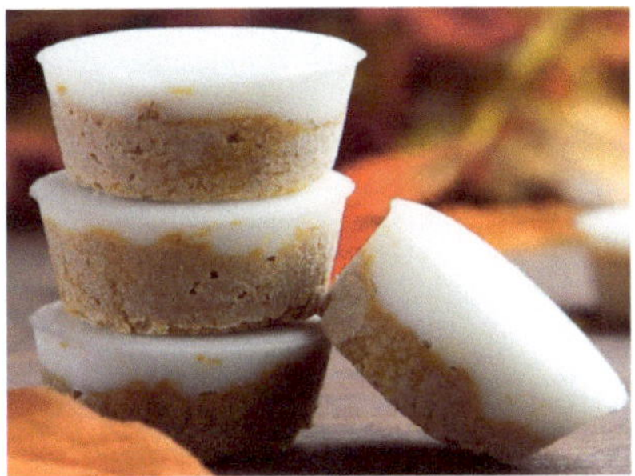

Ingredients:

- 200 grams long-shredded coconut (unsweetened)

- ½ cup coconut oil

- A pinch to ¼ tsp. of rock salt

- 25 drops of stevia extract (alcohol-free)

- 1 tbsp. ground cinnamon

- ¾ cup unsweetened pumpkin puree

- 1 and ½ tsp. ground ginger

- ¼ tsp. pure vanilla extract (alcohol-free)

- A pinch of ground cloves

- Optional ingredient: ¼ cup grass-fed collagen

Instructions:

1. Prepare a baking sheet then line it with mini-muffin silicone molds.

2. Process the coconut oil, shredded coconut, salt, and stevia in your food processor until the mixture is smooth enough.

3. Take around one-fourth cup of the coconut mix while leaving the remaining mix in your food processor. Add the other ingredients into the food processor then process until a smooth mixture is produced.

4. Divide this processed mixture into the mini-muffin cups arranged in a baking sheet. Press down until the mixture is completely flat. Top each cup with the coconut mixture you reserved earlier.

5. Store the baking sheet in your freezer and freeze before serving.

Nutritional Value: Calories – 219; Carbs – 6 grams; Protein – 3.6 grams; Fat – 182 grams

Blackberry and Coconut Fat Bomb

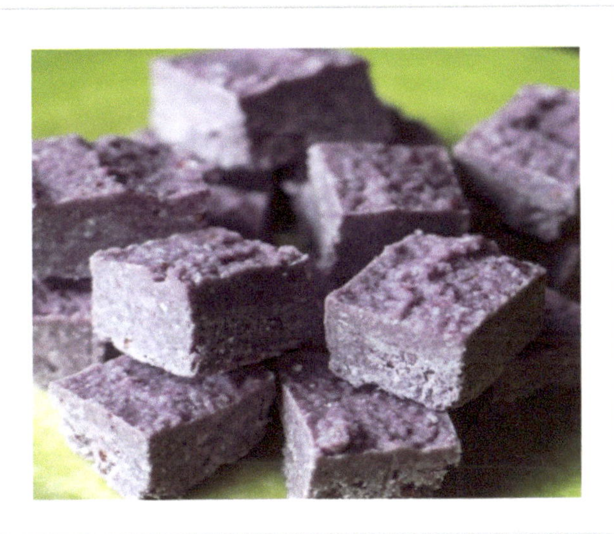

Ingredients:

- 1 cup each of coconut oil and coconut butter

- ½ cup frozen or fresh blackberries

- ¼ tsp. vanilla powder

- ½ tsp. stevia drops

- 1 tbsp. lemon juice

Instructions:

1. Put coconut oil, blackberries, and coconut butter in a pot. Set the pot over medium heat and heat the mixture for a few minutes.

2. Pour the coconut oil mixture into your food processor and add the remaining ingredients. Process until a smooth mixture is achieved.

3. Line a pan with parchment paper then spread the mixture out there. Store the pan in your fridge for a while until the mixture hardens or solidifies.

4.   After that, you can take it out of the container. Cut into squares.

5.   Store in your fridge again while covered before finally serving.

Nutritional Value: Calories – 170; Carbs – 3 grams; Protein – 1.1 gram; Fat – 18.7 grams

Lemon Curd Fat Bombs

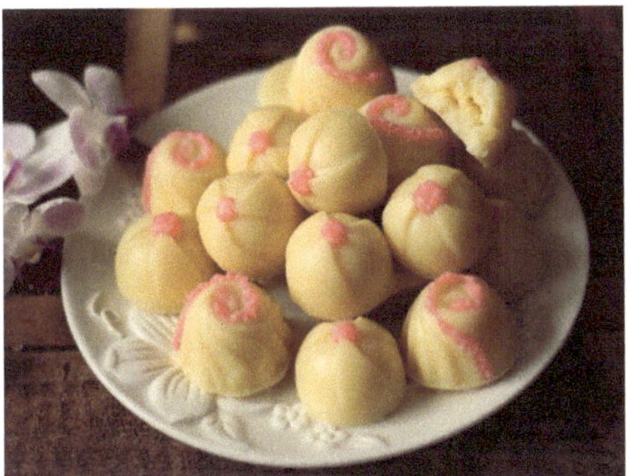

Ingredients for the coating:

- 2/3 cup Swerve confectioners

- 4-oz. edible cocoa butter

- ¼ tsp. Celtic sea salt

- 1 tsp. lemon extract

Ingredients for the filling:

- ½ cup lemon juice

- 1 cup Swerve

- 1 tbsp. lemon peel (finely grated)

- 8 tbsps. coconut oil

- 4 large eggs

Instructions:

1. Get a double boiler and put the cocoa butter in there. Set it over medium-high heat and heat until it fully melts. Stir in the natural sweetener, salt, and extracts.

2. Put the mixture in a truffle mold then allow it to cool down and solidify in your fridge.

3. Prepare the lemon curb filling by mixing together the natural sweetener, eggs, lemon peel, and lemon juice in a saucepan. Whisk to mix everything. Pour the coconut oil. Continue whisking while setting the pan over medium heat until it produces a thickened mixture.

4. Once done, use a strainer to pour this mixture into a medium-sized bowl. Put this bowl into another bowl, a larger one with ice water. Whisk it occasionally until you notice that the filling has cooled down completely.

5. Make the truffle. You can do that by removing the mold from your freezer or fridge first then filling it with the prepared lemon curd. Top it off with one layer of cocoa butter mixture. Return to your fridge and store it there to set.

Nutritional Value: Calories – 138; Carbs – 12 grams; Protein – 1 gram; Fat – 10 grams

Mocha Ice Bombs

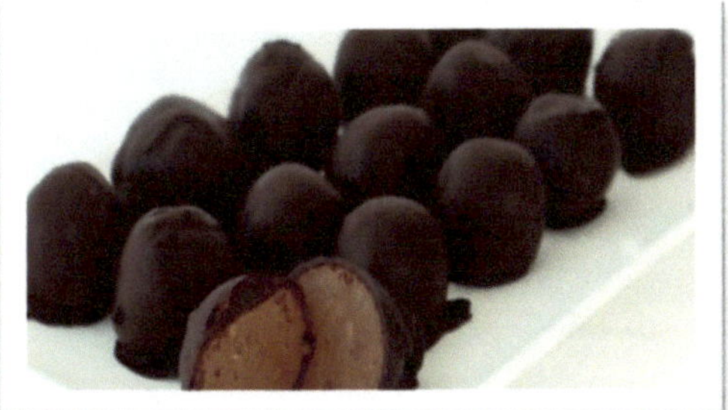

Ingredients:

- 240 grams mascarpone or cream cheese

- 2 tbsps. unsweetened cocoa

- 4 tbsps. powdered sweetener

- 60-ml chilled strong coffee

- 70 grams chocolate (melted)

- 28 grams cocoa butter (melted)

Instructions:

1. Add the chilled coffee into the mascarpone or cream cheese and put them in your food processor. Put the sweetener and cocoa, too. Pulse or blend the mixture until it becomes smooth.

2. To create the shape of the ice bomb, roll around 2 tablespoons of the prepared mixture then place in a plate or tray lined with parchment paper.

3. Prepare the coating by mixing the melted cocoa butter and chocolate together. Roll each prepared ice bomb into the coating then put back into the plate or tray.

4. Store in your freezer until set and serve.

Nutritional Value: Calories – 127; Carbs – 2.2 grams; Protein – 1.9 gram; Fat – 12.9 grams

Peanut Butter Fat Bombs

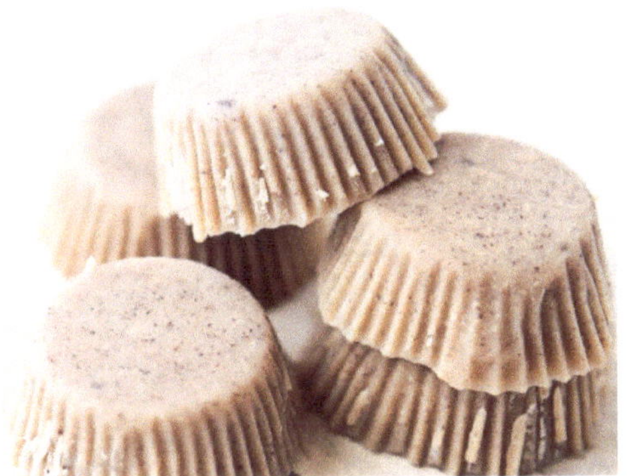

Ingredients:

- ¼ cup clean peanut butter

- ½ cup virgin coconut oil

- 1 tsp. pure vanilla extract

- 1 and ½ tsp. ground cinnamon

- Pure liquid stevia

Instructions:

1. Combine all the mentioned ingredients in a bowl with the help of a spoon.

2. Arrange cupcake liners/papers or mini-muffin papers in a baking tray. Pour around one tablespoon of the prepared mixture into the cupcake or mini-muffin paper. Put the baking tray in your freezer and store it there until the mixture solidifies.

3. Once it fully solidifies, take the fat bombs out of the tray then put them in a container or bag. Place them into the freezer again.

4. Serve it anytime you want.

Nutrition Value: Calories – 103; Carbs – 1 gram; Protein – 1 gram; Fat – 10 grams

Peppermint Mocha Fat Bombs

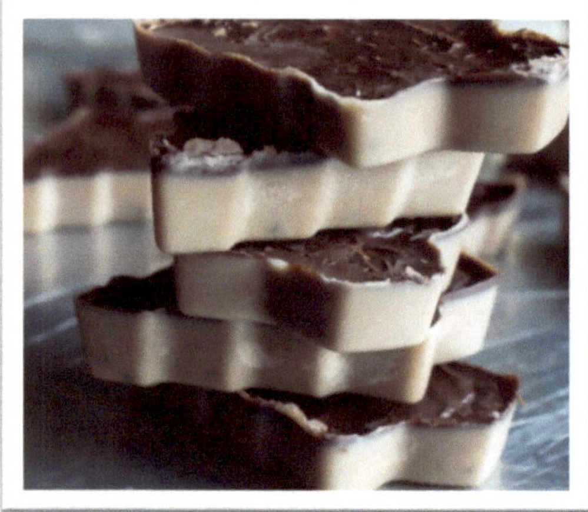

Ingredients:

- 3 tbsps. each of melted coconut oil and hemp seeds

- ¾ cup melted coconut butter

- 2 tbsps. organic cocoa powder

- ¼ tsp. peppermint extract

- 5 to 8 drops liquid stevia

- 2 tsps. of instant coffee powder

Instructions:

1. Mix the melted coconut butter, hemp seeds, peppermint extract, and 1 tbsp. of the coconut oil. Pour this mixture into molds, being careful that it fills around three-fourth of each mold.

2. Refrigerate until it becomes firm.

3. Mix the remaining melted coconut oil, stevia, instant coffee, and cocoa powder together. Drizzle this mixture over each solidified fat bomb.

4. Store in your fridge again until the fat bombs harden completely. After that, you can pop them out of their molds. Transfer them into an airtight container.

Nutritional Value: Calories – 121; Carbs – 4 grams; Protein – 2 grams; Fat – 11 grams

Keto Macaroon Fat Bombs

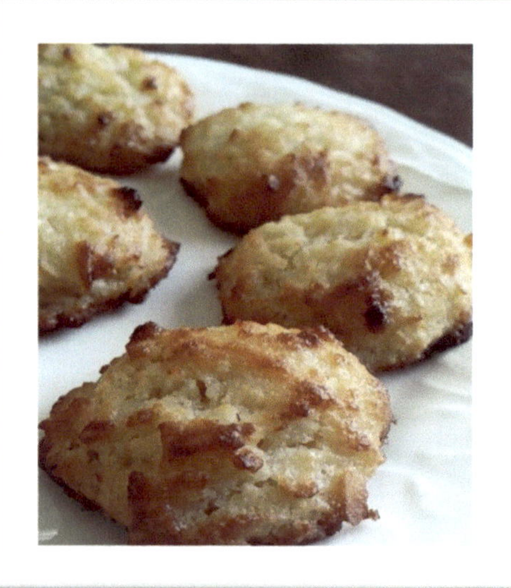

Ingredients:

- 1/2 cup shredded coconut

- ¼ cup almond flour

- 2 tbsps. Swerve

- 1 tbsp. each of coconut oil and vanilla extract

- 3 egg whites

Instructions:

1. Mix the almond flour, swerve, and coconut in a bowl first. Make sure that these ingredients are well-blended.

2. The next step is melting coconut oil in a pan. Pour the vanilla extract into it.

3. Chill a medium-sized bowl in your freezer. You will be using this to mount the egg whites.

4.   Pour the melted coconut oil over the flour mixture. Mix well.

5.   Once the bowl is chilled, put the egg whites in there. Whisk them until they become stiff.

6.   Put the egg whites gently into the flour mixture. Avoid over mixing, though.

7.   The next step is adding spoonfuls of the mixture into muffin cups or a cookie sheet. Bake in your oven until the macaroons begin to brown.

8.   You should then take them out of your oven. Allow the macaroons to cool before taking them out of the cookie sheet and serving.

Nutritional Value: Calories – 46; Carbs – 0.5 gram; Protein – 1.8 gram; Fat – 5 grams

Almond Butter Fat Bombs

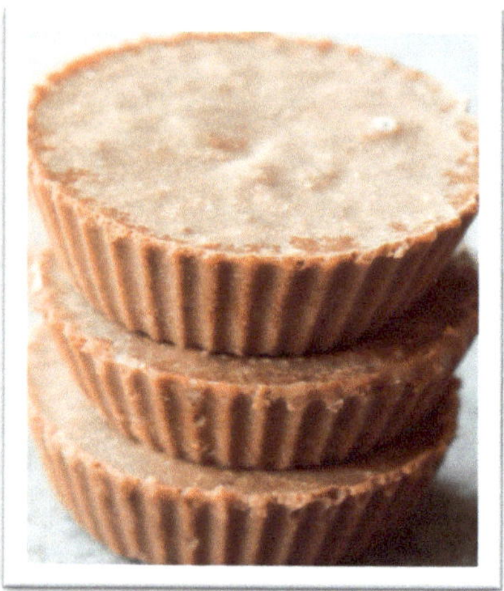

Ingredients:

- ¼ cup each of unrefined coconut oil and almond butter

- ¼ cup erythritol

- 2 tbsps. cacao powder

Instructions:

1. Mix coconut oil and almond butter in a medium-sized bowl.

2. Microwave this mixture for around thirty to forty-five seconds. Stir the mixture until it becomes smooth.

3. Add the cacao powder and erythritol into the mix. After that, you can start pouring it into silicone molds.

4. Store in your refrigerator until it becomes firm. Serve.

Nutritional Value: Calories – 189; Carbs – 3.6 grams; Protein – 3.2 grams; Fat – 19.1 grams

Nutty Coconut Fat Bombs

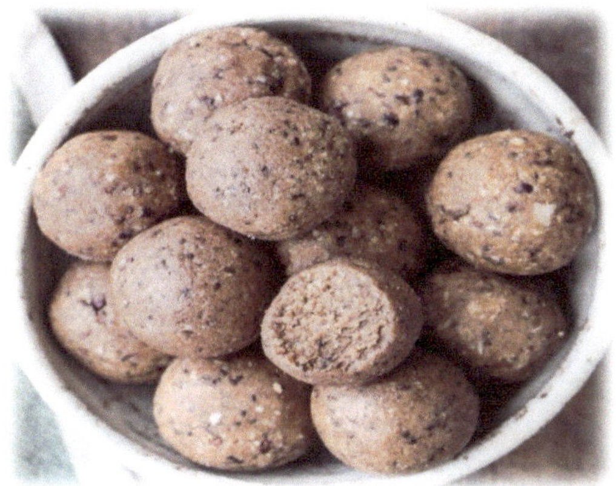

Ingredients:

- 1 and ½ cups walnut

- ¼ cup coconut butter

- ½ cup coconut (shredded)

- 2 tbsps. each of almond butter, chia seeds, hemp seeds, and flax meal

- 1 tsp. cinnamon

- 1 tbsp. maple syrup (optional)

- 2 tbsps. cacao nibs

- ½ tsp. vanilla bean powder

- ¼ tsp. kosher salt

Chocolate Drizzle Ingredients:

- ½ tsp. coconut oil

- 1 oz. unsweetened or bittersweet chocolate (chopped)

Instructions:

1. In your food processor's bowl, mix all the mentioned ingredients with the exception of the cacao nibs. Pulse the mixture for around one to two minutes or until the time when the mixture begins to break down. Continue processing until the oils are released slightly and the entire mix easily sticks together.

2. Divide the mixture evenly with the help of a cookie or tablespoon scoop. Start rolling the mixture into balls using your hands. Put the balls in a plate.

3. Prepare the chocolate drizzle. You can do that by using your microwave to melt the coconut oil and chocolate together for around thirty seconds to one minute. Drizzle this mixture over each ball.

4. Place in your fridge to make it firmer before serving.

Nutritional Value: Calories – 164; Carbs – 6 grams; Protein – 4 grams; Fat – 14 grams

Cherry and Chocolate Fat Bomb

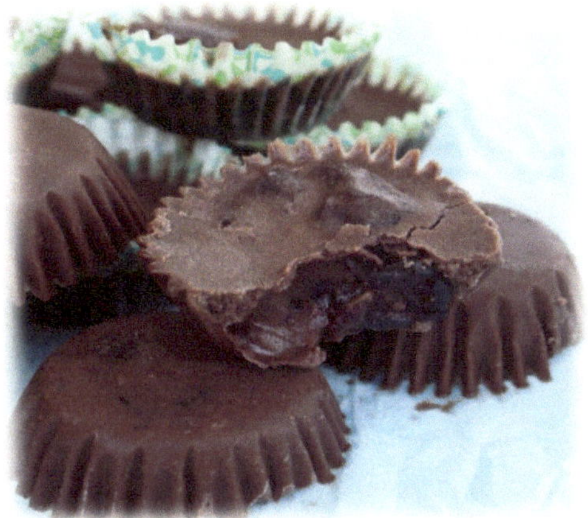

Ingredients:

- ¼ cup each of melted coconut butter and coconut oil

- 5 drops of Stevia

- 3 tbsps. cacao powder

- ¾ cup thawed frozen dark sweet cherries

- ½ tsp. each of vanilla extract and almond extract

Instructions:

1. Combine all the ingredients with the exception of the dark cherries.

2. Once you have thawed the frozen cherries, use a fork to mash them. Combine the cherries together with their juices into the chocolate mixture.

3. Spoon a tablespoonful of the mixture into an ice cube tray or mini-cupcake liner. Freeze it in your freezer before serving.

Nutritional Value: Calories – 67; Carbs – 2 grams; Fats – 6 grams

White Chocolate Fat Bomb

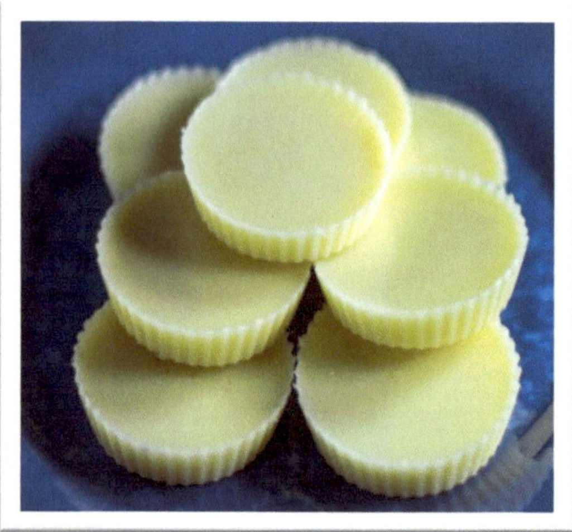

Ingredients:

- ¼ cup each of coconut oil and cocoa butter

- 10 drops of vanilla Stevia

Instructions:

1. Melt coconut oil and cocoa butter together in a double boiler or over low heat. Once done, you can take this mixture out of the heat.

2. Stir in the vanilla-flavored Stevia. Pour the mixture into molds.

3. Store in your fridge to chill until it hardens.

4. Remove from the molds then serve.

Nutritional Value: Calories – 125; Fat – 10 grams

Fudge Fat Bombs

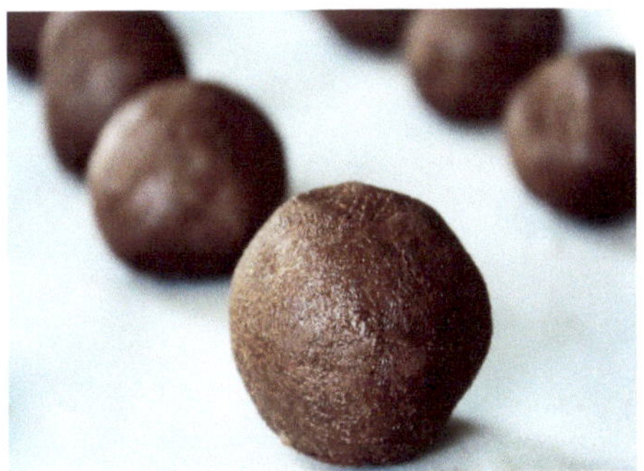

Ingredients:

- 1 cup each of coconut oil and almond butter

- 1/3 cup coconut flour

- ½ cup cocoa powder (unsweetened)

- ¼ tsp. powdered stevia

- Some pink Himalayan salt

Instructions:

1. Put a small-sized pot over medium heat. Combine coconut oil and almond butter there and allow the mixture to melt.

2. Stir in the dried ingredients and mix until fully combined. Let the mixture cool a bit. Do a taste test to figure out whether you need to add more sweetener.

3. Pour the mixture into a silicone mold and store the fat bombs in your freezer to solidify. Serve and enjoy.

Nutritional Value: Calories – 128; Carbs – 3.4 grams; Protein – 2 grams; Fat – 12

French Toast Fat Bomb

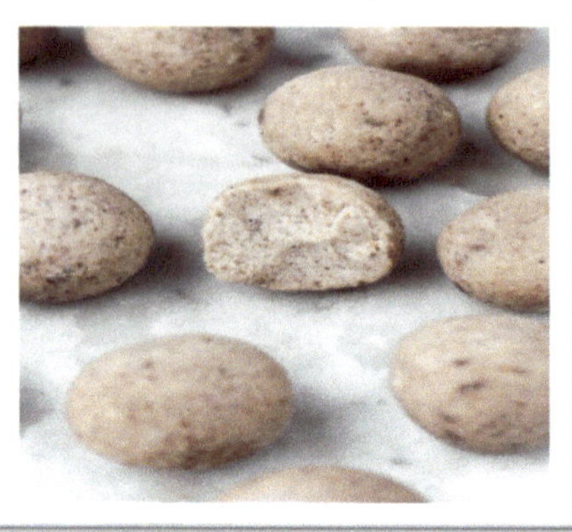

Ingredients:

- 8-oz. softened cream cheese

- ½ cup almond butter

- 1 stick softened unsalted butter

- 1/3 cup each of fruit sweetener and maple-flavored syrup

- ½ tsp. pure vanilla extract

- 1 tsp. maple extract

Instructions:

1. Mix all the mentioned ingredients in a bowl with the aid of your electric mixer. Freeze this mixture for a while.

2. After that, remove it from your fridge and create balls out of it. Use a parchment paper as a lining for the plate and put each fat bomb on top.

3. Put the fat bombs in your freezer again to achieve your desired firmness then serve.

Nutritional Value: Calories – 100; Carbs – 6. 9 grams; Protein – 1.9 grams; Fat – 9.5 grams

Jam and Peanut Butter Fat Bomb

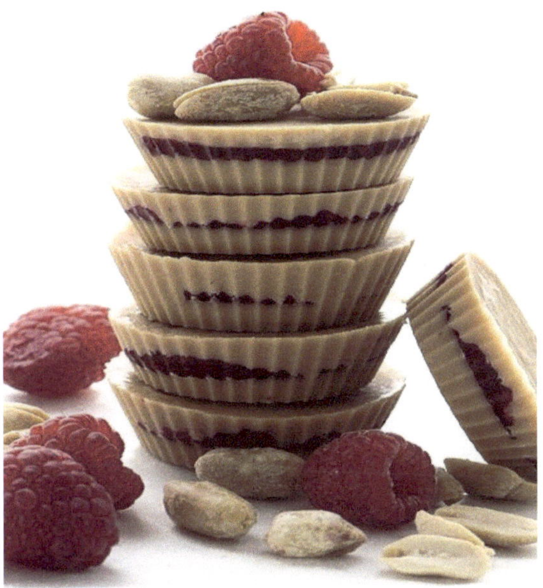

Ingredients:

- ¼ cup water

- ¾ cup raspberries

- 1 tsp. grass-fed gelatin

- 6-8 tbsps. swerve sweetener (powdered and divided)

- ¾ cup each of coconut oil and creamy peanut butter

Instructions:

1. Get a muffin pan then line it with around a dozen of parchment paper or silicone liners.

2. Mix water and raspberries and put the mixture in a medium-sized saucepan set over medium heat. Boil then reduce heat. Simmer it for around five minutes. Use a fork to mash the raspberries.

3. Add around two to four tablespoons of the powdered sweetener. This will be dependent on your preferred sweetness. Add the grass-fed gelatin. Let it cool for a bit while you prepare the mixture containing the peanut butter.

4. Combine coconut oil and peanut butter in a bowl, which is safe to use in a microwave. Cook it using high setting for around thirty to sixty seconds or until the mixture melts. Add the remaining powdered sweetener.

5. Divide half of the mixture containing peanut butter among the twelve cups or liners. Allow the mixture to firm up in your fridge for a few minutes. After that, you can pour the raspberry mixture over the cups. Use the remaining peanut butter mix to top of each cup.

6. Store in your fridge until ready to serve.

Nutritional Value: Calories – 223; Carbs – 4.52 grams; Protein – 3.84 grams; Fat – 21.77 grams

Cinnamon Roll Fat Bomb

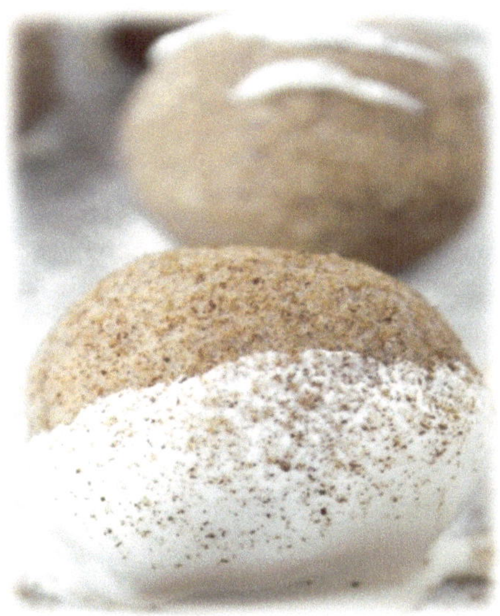

Ingredients:

- 8-oz. softened cream cheese

- ½ cup each of crunchy almond butter and softened butter

- 2 tsps. cinnamon

- ½ cup fruit sweetener

- 1 tsp. vanilla extract

For the frosting:

- 2 tsps. fruit sweetener

- 1 and ½ oz. softened cream cheese

- ¼ tsp. vanilla extract

- 1 tbsp. heavy whipping cream

Instructions:

1. Mix all the required ingredients for the fat bomb in a bowl with the help of your electric mixer. Store in your fridge for a few minutes.

2. Get a plate and use parchment paper to line it. Take the bowl containing the mixture out of your refrigerator and form balls out of it. Arrange the fat bombs on top of the plate lined with parchment paper.

3. Let the fat bombs harden a bit while you make the frosting. Just mix all the frosting ingredients in a bowl with the help of an electric mixer. Once done, you can take the bombs out of your freezer and frost.

4. Serve.

Nutritional Value: Calories – 103; Carbs – 6.5 grams; Protein – 2 grams; Fat – 10.3 grams

Conclusion

Keto fat bombs are indeed among the most flavorful recipes that you can make if you want to enjoy delicious snacks or meal replacements. What's even better about them is that they are easy to prepare. In fact, the majority of the keto fat bomb recipes in this book can be prepared in just ten minutes.

You also have the option of making either savory or sweet fat bombs depending on what you really prefer in terms of taste. Start making fat bombs and including them in your daily routines now and you will notice their effectiveness in making you feel energized while also filling you, thereby lessening your cravings.

-- Rick Elliot

www.ingramcontent.com/pod-product-compliance
Lightning Source LLC
Chambersburg PA
CBHW040301240726
48664CB00006B/1334